Men's Fashion

Basic Fashion Tips on How to Dress Enviably Manly

David Prince

Copyright © David Prince, 2018

Disclaimer

Contents

The Complacency Already Existing in Most Men's Fashion

Let's face it; fashion can make all the difference in the world. It is an integral part of self-presentation that most men don't pay much attention to and it is quite surprising the level of satisfaction some men show even when there's apparently an aberration in their dress sense. There's a famous saying that, "How you dress is the same way you will be addressed." This saying is not only accurate but has proven beyond reasonable doubts over time that a man's dress sense says a lot in telling who exactly he is, it explains in totality what his personality is, it sharpens people's thoughts of a man and creates a big picture in their memory.

Fashion isn't overrated, and it is beauteous when men with excellent dress sense are seen showcasing fashion in their own way. Most men don't even bother about fashion anymore, and it is saddening. The complacency noticed is numerous too.

Seeing a man who is ignorant about fashion tips sends a message. Seeing a slim man on a baggy or loose trouser can be demeaning as it indicates a disconnected look. Seeing a man going for a function requiring formal attires wearing a white tie on white jackets or long vests is awkward. Seeing a man who is chubby on small clothing is clearly against standards, fitness is a priority indeed, but fitness shouldn't be mistaken for small clothing. Seeing a man wearing pleather instead of leather shows low quality. Seeing a man on casual wears with too many designer labels makes the whole outfit look less attractive. Dressing too flashy isn't necessary, make it simple and smart!

Understanding the need to look good, trying to brace up to learn something new about fashion, focusing on basic stuff about fashion, getting a sensible wardrobe function, trying out new styles, showcasing beautiful colors in dressings; are all perfect for enhancing men's fashion. You bet!

It's not a rumor that fashion isn't all about the dresses alone but also matching the dresses with classy and exquisite bags, quality wristwatches and shoes, as well as other combinations that give a soothing presence.

"Being perfectly well-dressed gives one a tranquility that no religion can bestow."

—Ralph Waldo Emerson

Without doubts, most men have been denied many responsibilities due to their ignorance and complacency to fashion, and this makes the subject of men fashion an expedient one to address to teach unsuspecting men what it takes to dress like the man that everyone wants to be associated with. Fashion is everything, so remain classy!

"The style of studied nonchalance is the psychological triumph of grace over order."

—G. Bruce Boyer, Fashion Editor

What A Man's Wardrobe Should Look Like

(Types of Wears and Compartmentalization of the Different Types of Wears)

A man's wardrobe is directly proportional to his sense of fashion. It is indubitable that a man should have his closet stocked with a variety of wears, accessories and clothing materials. This gives an entire insight into his personality and what he thinks like. Different types of wears fit for different kinds of occasions making it necessary for a man to have a fully equipped wardrobe. It is delightful to know that each piece of clothing should complement other forms of dressing.

You should note that "a man who ignores his wardrobe is at his own risk." as a man's wardrobe obviously dictates his outlook and that outlook speaks louder than words. It's a good practice for a man to constantly check his clothes to discard the old and bad clothes, clean clothes that are stained, fix the fixable clothes and ultimately put in an extra effort to make his closet unique.

Without question, a man's wardrobe should contain the following:

- White Shirts
- A few Corporate Suits
- Blazers
- Bomber Jackets
- Underwear of Different Colors and Designs
- Chinos
- Flannels
- Sports Coats
- Track Suit
- Jeans
- Chino Shorts
- Denim Jackets
- Sweaters

- T-Shirts
- Polo Shirts

Proper arrangement and compartmentalization of these wears are what makes the wardrobe of a real man appealing. They also aid in the easy selection of wears and help in making better choices to suit your taste. Of course, other dressing accessories should spice up a man's closet, and these include leather belts, pleasant colognes, and wristwatches to mention but a few.

What Should You Wear, When?

Apparently, there are so many activities to get involved in, and they all require unique dresses and especially combinations to make a man look apt for the right occasion. A man needs to be trendy to make any sense fashion-wise. So, it's not all about the wearing of clothes, but knowing how best to combine wears with regards to their type, texture, colors, etc. I will be mentioning a few occasions and the best dress combination that should be worn to look presentable enough for the event.

Work

The type of work you do goes a long way in determining how you dress for it. For a corporate office job, you need to be in your shirt and pants with the shirt tucked into the pant. Your pant should be of a neutral color (like black, grey, brown, etc.) while you change the color of your shirt. And of course, you don't want to forget your tie; basically, you should wear a long tie and not a bow. You could put some sauce on your corporate dressing by wearing a suit; more respect is placed on your name with that. Basically, your workplace should dictate your dressing; so, do not bother much, just ensure the right combination and you're good to go.

"A well-tied tie is the first serious step in life."

—Oscar Wilde, Poet

Weddings

The dress code should have been explicitly stated in the invitation, and if it is not, it is pertinent to contact the event host for the dress codes.

For weddings where the black tie is chosen by the event hosts, that alone sends a message that it's all about low-key personalization and black tuxedos, white shirts, black bow ties and leather shoes can make a perfect combo.

For weddings where you're asked to dress casually, keep in mind that shorts, denim, or t-shirt are no-nos. You still need to look sharp.

For weddings where no dress code is dictated, this is indeed an opportunity to do your thing neatly and fantastically but take cautions, so it won't seem like you've overshadowed the day's event.

Cocktail Parties

Wearing a formal shirt or a regularly worn shirt to a cocktail party seems awkward as a cocktail party is an excellent avenue for merriment and relaxation. Get your jackets and trousers well ironed and ready to roll.

Get your face pampered, visit the barber's salon and get new hair products as all these will contribute to making you look fabulous.

Wearing slacks with improper lengths and ill fittings are solely inappropriate. Figure-hugging blazers and fitted trousers are a good match for cocktail parties. Keep it simple, look comfortable and smart!

Dinner parties

Think about what type of dinner party it is to serve as a guide in making decisions. Dark denim, chinos, blazers, etc. are appropriate for dinner parties.

Job Interviews

First of all, make inquiries about the company's dress code on their website, and you must keep in mind that your dressings should spell out confidence as the very first assessment is based on appearances and how smart you look. Tidy up your fingernails, your facial hairs should be appropriately taken care of, and your socks should match the color of your pants. If wearing sweaters, it should be worn with a button-down shirt.

"Clothes don't make a man, but clothes have got many a man a good job." —Herbert Harold Vreeland, Academic

---

Funerals

Funerals are emotional occasions, and it is apparently not a place to show off as a fashionista. Too many accessories are inappropriate. Understanding the atmospheric condition of the location is also essential as you won't want to sweat during summer or catch a cold during Spring. Of course, you should mostly be on all black, the weather should then determine if you'll need a suit or just your shirt will suffice.

Casual Setting

Hanging out with friends, family, or visiting a neighbor? You still don't want to look shabby jut because it's a casual setting. Wear your T-shirt or Polo Shirt with your jeans or chinos pants/shorts stylishly. You want to feel very comfortable in a casual setting, so something light and that allows air onto your body is a great choice.

Basic Color Combination Rules

Some of our life procedures seem to have been defined and perfected by mother nature. From being a pleasurable kid who derives so much joy in wearing clothes that exhibits beautiful colors to learning the identification of colors gradually and how best not to look stupid. It's all a part of a process nature has subconsciously placed in us over the years.

Knowing how to match colors is of great importance as colors spark emotions in people who assess your dressing. Colors are encompassing, and colors have indeed played a significant role in the beautification of the universe itself. So why not your dressing as a real man? Never allow anyone to shade your dress sense because of a whack color combo.

There are many color codes to follow when making one's choice of wears and getting your color codes and combos right goes a long way in showing how excellent your knowledge of fashion is.

Warm colors are known to create a feeling of happiness, passion, and enthusiasm. On the other hand, cool colors bring about calmness and peace. However, did you know that combining warm and cool colors may result in aesthetic errors?

The color theory is to be well understood as it plays a significant role in choosing what to wear and it should also serve as an initial platform for fashion beginners to learn the right color combinations.

Red, blue and yellow are primary colors, and the mix of red and yellow will give orange, the mix of blue and red will give violet, the combination of blue and yellow will give green. Hence, making orange, violet and green secondary colors. Tertiary colors are gotten when secondary colors and primary colors are mixed together. The arrangements of these hues on the color wheel make choosing colors easier. Wearing an outfit that consists of blue and orange makes an excellent combination.

Selecting colors like blue and orange, green and red is very much pleasant for wears varying on the level of saturation and brightness considered. Imagine wearing a cloth that has blue tints and orange with exquisite shoes.

Selecting colors like red, yellow and blue with brilliant levels of saturation and brightness spells out how classy one is.

Selecting colors like blue and orange to be mixed with red and green may at first look a bit off but will exhibit creativity in the long run.

It is also advisable to focus on neutral colors like black, white, gray, brown – to mention but a few – when choosing your wears. These colors are basically foundations for any output. You could try these on as a mix with more eye-catchy and bolder colors in a bid to experiment and look great. These colors mostly go great with pants as almost any other bolder color of the upper wear will combine well with these pant colors regardless of your skin tone or the occasion in question.

"To achieve the nonchalance which is absolutely necessary for a man, one article at least must not match."

—Hardy Amies, Couturier

Why don't you try out some nice color combinations on your own, then stare at the mirror to see if it looks appealing? If it does, then go for it!

Following one's mind increases your confidence level, and confidence in anything and everything you do matters a lot.

Other Tips Men Should Take Note of When Dressing

Apparently, complementing one's dressing is of great importance and some guidelines should be followed. Reading fashion and style books is expedient as it is a good start for a man who is looking forward to upgrading his style.

Shopping with friends is another good styling tip as your friends will tell you exactly how you look like in the outfit you intend buying and their opinions will be with fair judgments as it will be different from that of the store attendants who are majorly interested in making sales.

A man should always dress like his schedules for the day might change, and his attention may be needed at another location at any other time of the day like a restaurant or a club, or even a reasonably formal meeting. "If I am unable to go back home and change, is this presentable to wear to other possible location?" That's a good question to ask yourself as a man before choosing your wears. For instance, you know you have a date in the evening but can't go home from work to change before the date, you want to wear removable top layers in case unexpected happenings like lending your jacket or shirt to the damsel comes up.

Unarguably, a man should always clean his clothes regularly as stains are easily noticed in public; your wallets should also be cleaned too. Most men don't pay attention to cleaning or changing their wallets but imagine dressing enviably to a supermarket to get some groceries, and your wallet looks all messy when you're about to pay. How embarrassing is that?

Involve in workouts and exercises as much as possible to help build that body shape that makes clothes look great on you.

Wearing a cologne isn't a bad idea after all as it complements one's dressing significantly too.

More so, taking comprehensive care of the skin is also necessary as the aim is to dress the entire body and look ravishing. You can also complement your dressing with pieces of jewelry like rings, male or unisex chains, etc.

Getting well-designed backpacks is also an excellent way to go as it exhibits one's superabundant knowledge of what fashion is all about.

Pay proper attention to how you wear and combine your casual wears too because they also tell how fashionable or not you are.

Practice rolling up your shirtsleeves in a couple of ways as it excites when properly done.

Too much graphics on clothes is usually a turn off for men in a formal setting. Clothes that have the designer's logo printed too boldly is also bad for a stylish general outlook.

Finally, never forget that the aim is to choose quality over quantity!

Final Words

Fashion sense is usually an expression of who a person, especially a man, really is. And there's nothing so complicated about having an exquisite and enviable dress sense as a man. I want to believe I have alleviated your ignorance or worries to an extent with this short book and now you can stand tall enough to start making the right choices with your clothes, cloth accessories, as well as color combinations that make everyone commend your command as a man. Learn new ways to upgrade your dressing styles and follow your heart at most times. Pick the right clothes for the right occasions and remember never to over-dress. Keep it simple and smart and earn the respect of whoever beholds your magnificence.

Remember,

"Style is the perfection of a point of view."—
Richard Eberhart, Poe

I hope that this book has provided value to you and benefitted you on your fashion journey. If so, an honest review of the book would be very appreciated.

www.ingramcontent.com/pod-product-compliance
Lightning Source LLC
Chambersburg PA
CBHW051240250726
48656CB00003B/1052